S.T.E.P.S Towards Organic Living
Non-Toxic Living on a Budget

Shari Ware

shariware.com

Shari's Other Books

Fat to Fabulous: Diet Free Weight Loss for Real Women

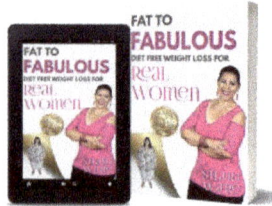

Healthy! Beautiful Inside & Out

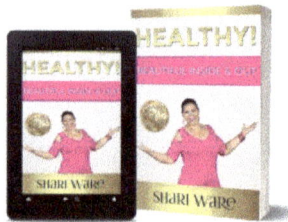

Reclaim Your Inner Goddess

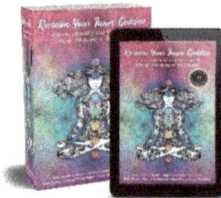

Grab Your Copies At: shariware.com/books

Before you get started, watch this welcome video (shariware.com/STOLWelcome) to help you get the most out of this book.

This book comes with a downloadable workbook filled with action steps to help you create **Your Organic Blueprint** as you progress through the book. Go to shariware.com/STOLWorkbook to download the workbook prior to reading this book or scan the QR code below.

You'll find the corresponding page number of the workbook listed at each action step.

ISBN: 978-0-6485048-4-9

Acknowledgments

I'd like to thank my amazing daughter Nataasjia and her furbaby Lulu. Nataasjia is my biggest cheerleader and (mostly) humours my "multiple convincer" personality, albeit with a lot of sighs and eyerolls! I am so blessed and grateful that despite being a millennial, she is happily on this journey with me and that she brought her furbaby Lulu along for the ride. I love you both so much.

Love always, Mumma Bear/Nene

Xoxo

Contents

Introduction

Do you want to make the transition to a healthier lifestyle but struggle to do so? Does the word "organic" give you visions of money burning a hole through your pocket? Have you tried and given up because it seemed like a mammoth task, and you were completely overwhelmed? If this is you, then you're in the right place!

Firstly, let me tell you how excited I am that you are here reading this book. My mission in life is to help people just like you make healthy changes in their lives by focusing on doing a little better every day.

It's not about being perfect; it's just about being a little better than we were yesterday.

I call it the B ME Movement - Better Me Every Day!

If you love that and it speaks to you, we're on the same page!

The purpose of this book is to help you take the pain and overwhelm out of switching to organic. I promise you that it IS possible! Whether you're a young adult, an older adult, or in between; whether you're an established family, or you're pregnant with your first child; a couple, single or a pet owner; no matter where you are on your organic journey – this book will help.

I know how you feel because I used to be just like you. Back in 2010, I embarked on a weight LOSS journey, which you can read about in my first book **Fat to Fabulous – Diet Free Weight Loss for Real Women.** At some point it turned into a weight RELEASE

1

journey and, finally, it turned into a HEALTH journey, which you can read about in my second book Healthy! Beautiful Inside & Out.

Back in 2016, as my health journey continued, I became aware that for my BEST health, I needed to switch to organic, or BETTER choices. I had made a lot of great changes already, but up until this point in time, I had no conscious knowledge of there being anything wrong with mainstream food or other products.

But as always, when I'm ready for the next part of my journey, the path opens up ahead of me and I'm given the information I need to take the first step on that path. Even if it's not where I thought I wanted to go...

When the organic path opened up ahead of me, it took me a while to actually take the first step. At first, I struggled with the belief that I couldn't afford to switch to organic. I felt like I didn't have enough time to make the switch, to travel to different places to get different items instead of being able to go to one grocery store to get everything I needed, to do the necessary research, to read labels.

I was totally overwhelmed by all the things that I felt I needed to change. It felt so hard, and I felt like it would never be DONE!

Despite all that, I eventually took the first step, and then another, and then another, and here we are today. I have switched so many things to organic in my life and continue to do so. And do you want to know the most awesome thing? Out of all the negative beliefs I had in the beginning, I was only right about one of them. I bet you wanna know which one? I'll tell you a little later...

So, if you haven't got the gist by now, let me make it clear that I absolutely GET it! I know what you're going through, I know how you're feeling, and I know that this book will help.

Here's how.

In Chapter 1, you are going to get started on your WHY. You can do ANYTHING when you have what I call WHY Power! WHY organic? WHY make the switch?

In Chapter 2, you'll learn mindset tools, tips, and strategies to make the transition to organic painless and effortlessly easy. You may not believe that's possible, but by the end of the chapter, you'll have a whole different perspective.

In Chapters 3 and 4, you're going to create Your Organic Blueprint which will be your personalized plan to follow step-by-step to your destination. You'll decide what your destination is and then assess where you're at currently on your journey to a healthier lifestyle.

Chapter 5 will give you practical, budget-friendly tools, tips, and strategies to navigate the maze, while Chapter 6 will give you a crash course on reading food labels. You'll be amazed at the nasties hidden in plain sight!

Chapter 7 is all about acknowledging and celebrating your organic journey and in lucky Chapter 8, you'll find my top suggestions and resources to help you fast track your journey to make the entire process quicker and easier.

There will be small action steps for you to take along the way and you'll be given all the tools and resources you need. You'll get the most out of this book by engaging actively and DOING rather than just reading. So, before you get started, grab your downloadable workbook that you can print that includes all the activities in the book.

You may be tempted to skip the activities, but I promise you that if you give yourself the gift of doing them, you'll discover things deep inside yourself you never knew were there.

Ready to get started?

Let's go!

Your Organic Blueprint Action Step

It's time for your first action step! Before you start, watch this short video [(shariware.com/YOBASIntro)](shariware.com/YOBASIntro) to get some tips on how to get the most out of this action step.

On **Page 4** of the downloadable workbook, answer the following questions:

- Think about how you feel about the difficulty of transitioning to organic before reading this book. On a scale of 1-10 (where 1 is extremely difficult and 10 is totally easy), how would you rate your current feelings?
- Write down three words to describe how you currently feel about the difficulty of transitioning to organic.

66

"You don't have to be perfect. Just focus on doing a little better each day."

-shari ware

Chapter 1
Organic: Why Should You Make the Switch?

So, why organic? Why does it matter and why should you make the switch? What does "organic" even mean and what are the basics that you need to know? These are all great questions!

Why Organic?

The food we have in the 21st century is not the same as the food we had just a century ago and back through the ages. In modern times, mainstream food is mass produced, highly processed, genetically modified, and has nasty chemicals added to it.

Primary producers of fresh produce use insecticides, pesticides, herbicides, fungicides, rodenticides, and several other kinds of "cides" to kill pests. Primary producers of meat feed their animals unhealthy grains to fatten them up and pump them full of antibiotics. Sounds tasty, right?!

You've heard the saying "you are what you eat"? If you're eating mainstream food, you're eating a whole bunch of nasty substances which eventually take a toll on your health, if it hasn't already.

What Does "Organic" Mean?

When we use the term "organic", we're talking about foods and products that have been farmed or produced as naturally as possible. The way that our food used to be produced – free from nasty chemicals, additives, preservatives, antibiotics, and genetic modifications.

Sometimes it's labelled "organic"; sometimes it's not. We'll go deeper into that a bit later, but for now, let's look at *why* you should make the switch.

Why Should You Switch to Organic?
There are three important reasons...

Better health
It's better for your health, your family's health, and your pets' health. Mainstream food and products are full of toxic and carcinogenic chemicals, artificial colours and preservatives, hormone disrupters, petroleum (yes, in your food! – we'll cover this later), heavy metals, antibiotics, and much more.

As if that isn't bad enough, mainstream food doesn't contain the nutrient density that organically produced food does. Studies show that the nutrient density in conventionally produced food has dropped by up to 76% since 1940. *Wowsers*! But studies also show nutrient density to be 25% higher in organic food than conventionally produced food. This means that organically produced food contains more vitamins, minerals, antioxidants, and phytochemicals, and all the rest of the good stuff for each calorie consumed.

Boosts the Local Economy
We'll discuss this in detail later, but when you're looking for organic, fresh food, you're likely buying from local farmers. This supports local small businesses which are the backbone of communities.

Helps the Environment
Mainstream farming practices involve releasing a myriad of chemicals into the environment, polluting the soil, waterways, and wildlife. Organic farmers use natural methods such as

rotation of crops, manure, and composting for pest control and fertilization.

Organic products also have much higher standards when it comes to animal welfare. Organically reared animals are raised in significantly better conditions and aren't pumped full of antibiotics and growth hormones, unlike mainstream farmed animals.

We're not just talking about what we eat either. Going back to the beginning of this chapter, I mentioned that "you are what you eat", but you're not just what YOU eat. You're also what you EAT eats. You're what you put ON your body. You're the air you breathe. You're what's in your environment and you're the thoughts you think.

Did you see that last one coming? Many people don't realise the impact that their thoughts have on their health, but your thoughts have a massive impact.

No matter where you are on your organic journey—the very beginning or part way through—there can be a LOT of things to think about, to assess, and to change. It can be overwhelming, and it can feel very difficult to do. In fact, it can even seem impossible. But I assure you that it's not.

In the next chapter, you'll learn how to make the transition painless and easy, but before we get to that, I want you to answer the following question:

WHY is it important for you to make this change?

Your Organic Blueprint Action Step

On **Page 5** of your downloadable workbook, write down the reasons WHY it's important for you to switch to organic.

> " "When you have massive WHY power, you don't NEED will power!"

-shari ware

Chapter 2
Reframing: Creating a Painless & Effortlessly Easy Transition

I can feel your disbelief...painless and effortlessly easy transition? That's not even possible, is it? Yes, it is! This chapter is all about how you can make the switch to organic in a way that's easy, sustainable and—dare I suggest it— sometimes even fun!

This chapter is all about mindset and it's the longest chapter because it's important that you have all the tools, tips, and strategies you need to build a strong foundation.

Later, we'll be covering practical tips, tools, and strategies for the actual physical transition. But you can't make the physical transition if you don't first make the mental transition. So let's dive in!

WHY Power!
In Chapter 1, we started to delve into your WHY and I included a quote: "When you have massive WHY Power, you don't NEED will power!"

This is something that I learned from my own weight loss journey. I lost 100kg naturally and the reason why I was finally able to do it after years of trying was because I found what I call my WHY Power!

One day, the scales finally tipped (pun not intended, but funny anyway) in the right direction and I was able to make the changes I needed to, one at a time, until I reached my goal.

Although I was grateful for it at the time, I didn't realise exactly what had happened until a couple of years later when I was listening to an audiobook called *The Secret Code of Success* by Noah St John. In it, Noah says, "*You can never solve a Why-To problem with a How-To solution.*"

That was an a-ha! moment for me, let me tell you! So, what does it mean?

Let's say you're trying to lose weight, but it doesn't matter how hard you try, you just can't seem to do it. You *really* want to lose the weight, but you can't make the changes you need to see results. It's not that you don't know WHAT to do or HOW to do it. Even if you don't know ALL the steps, you at least know one or two that would get you moving in the right direction, but you don't take them.

Why? Because for anything that you do in life, you have reasons WHY TO do them and reasons WHY NOT to do them and if the WHY NOTs outweigh the WHY TOs, then it doesn't matter how hard you try, you won't succeed.

You may not be conscious of your WHY NOTs, but they are there, deep in your subconscious. Even if you make some progress, eventually you'll self-sabotage and fail.

It's like we all have a set of those scales that have a plate on either side and when you add or take away weight from either side, they become unbalanced. If you want to succeed at whatever you're trying to achieve, your WHY TOs MUST outweigh your WHY NOTs.

This is why we started to delve into your WHY in the first chapter and why you're going to take a deeper dive in this chapter. Your

WHY Power is one of the elements that will help you make the switch to organic painless and effortless.

Anything is easier when you have a big enough WHY! At the end of this chapter, there will be a very special action step that will help you uncover the deep reason WHY you want to make the switch to organic.

The S.T.E.P.S Formula

It's time for me to introduce you to my unique framework called the S.T.E.P.S Formula. Drum roll please!

Most people have heard of SMART Goals, which are great. But if you don't know, it stands for **S**pecific, **M**easureable, **A**chieveable, **R**ealistic, **T**ime-Bound. I used to use SMART Goals, but I still struggled to succeed. And it was FRUSTRATING! I eventually realized that SMART Goals work best when you have the habits already created. But what happens when you don't? We need to find a way to make it easier in that scenario.

Introducing the S.T.E.P.S Formula! Ta-dah!

- **S**mall
- **T**imely
- **E**asy
- **P**leasurable
- **S**ustainable

Small

This is where a lot of people set themselves up for failure. Sometimes even when you think you've set yourself a small goal, it can still be too big. It's not that you can't have big goals – you absolutely can and it's highly recommended. But a goal is where you want to be, and it will take a series of steps to get there.

14

Most people set a big goal and then work their way towards it, but if it's too big and it seems like you're not making the progress you want, what usually happens? You give up. Which is totally understandable. The issue is not the size of the goal, it's the strategy used to achieve it. This is especially true if the habits needed to achieve the goal aren't yet formed. We'll be talking about the science behind habits soon, but for now, just know that it's important to break your big goal up into "mini goals" and that it's essential that you start small.

How small? There is NO start too small. It's better to underpromise and overdeliver. You'll give yourself a quick win, which will give you the motivation to keep moving forward.

Timely
Put a realistic timeframe around your goals and be open to the timeframe being flexible. You're aiming to make progress and any progress is good progress.

Easy
Yes, I said easy. How often have you had a picture in your head of how something is "supposed" to be and aimed for that exact picture, no matter how hard it was? Did you always succeed or did you fail sometimes? Have you told yourself in the past that you just have to "try harder"?

Instead of telling yourself to "try harder", ask yourself, "How can I make this easier?"

Just because you have a picture in your head of what something is supposed to look like, doesn't mean it has to be that way, and when you open yourself up to there being a different way and ask yourself how you can make it easier, you'll find what you're looking for.

15

When you're making a change in your life, the easier it is to do, the better. It's not a cop out either...it's SMART!

Pleasurable

This one is pretty self-explanatory, but it's important to emphasise that if the change you're trying to make is NOT pleasurable, please choose something else. If you're looking to make lifestyle changes to improve your health, you're generally not looking to make those changes for a week or a month or a year. You're planning on making those changes for the rest of your life, right? So, why would you choose to do something that you dislike for the rest of your life? That's unhealthy and defeats the whole purpose of making the change in the first place.

There are a myriad of different ways to make those changes, so find a strategy that you truly enjoy. Again, that's not a cop out...that's SMART!

Sustainable

This is also important for the same reason we discussed above. If you're looking to make a lifestyle change, it's not for a season, it's for a lifetime, so it absolutely has to be something you can sustain.

Ask yourself the question, "Will I like doing this for the rest of my life?" If you get any negative feelings, look for something else to change. It doesn't mean it will be off the table forever, it's just not right for you right now.

The Science Behind Habits

When you make something a habit, you do it automatically without even thinking about it, making it easy. Transitioning to healthier choices is going to be a lot easier if you approach it from the perspective of creating a series of habits that serve you.

Popular belief is that it takes 21 days to form a habit. This is not actually entirely correct and it's the reason why a lot of us regress after we think we've successfully created a new habit. Based on a study conducted by Phillippa Lally, a health psychology researcher at the University College London, which was published in the European Journal of Social Psychology, it can take anywhere from 18 to 254 days to create a new habit.

In most cases, it takes more than eight weeks to create a new habit and if you're looking for the average length of time, it takes exactly 66 days, which is over three times more than the common belief.

No wonder so many of us find ourselves back at square one just when we thought we had it all sorted!

Despite this, it is possible to create habits in 5-7 days. Did you know that there is a science behind habit formation? When you know the science behind it, it makes it so much easier to create healthy habits.

Habits consist of four components:

- The **TRIGGER** or CUE
- Which triggers the **DESIRE**
- To **BEHAVE** in a certain way
- Which gives us a **REWARD**

Each element is important and by changing one or more of them, you can either create a habit that serves you or stop a habit that doesn't.

If you want to stop a non-serving habit, you can:

- HIDE the TRIGGER or CUE
- Make the DESIRE UGLY or UNDESIRABLE
- Make it HARD to BEHAVE in the undesired way
- Make the REWARD UNSATISFACTORY

For instance, imagine you have a habit of checking your social media every ten minutes. You've realized that it's seriously affecting your productivity and you want to stop. You could:

- HIDE the TRIGGER or CUE by turning off all notifications on your devices and putting your phone out of sight when you're working.
- Make the DESIRE UGLY or UNDESIRABLE by putting your phone in another room or somewhere you have to spend time and considerable effort to go and retrieve it when you want it.
- Make it HARD to BEHAVE in the undesired way by turning the data off on your phone when you're not supposed to be on social media.
- Make the REWARD UNSATISFACTORY by compiling a list of the negative impacts of undisciplined use of social media and put it where you can see it easily.

If you want to create a habit that serves you, you can:

- Make the TRIGGER or CUE VISIBLE
- Make the DESIRE ATTRACTIVE
- Make it EASY to BEHAVE in the desired way
- Make the REWARD SATISFYING

For example, imagine that you wanted to create a meditation habit. You could:

- Make the TRIGGER or CUE VISIBLE by creating a special area for it.

18

- Make the DESIRE ATTRACTIVE by putting things that you love in the special area that makes you want to spend time there.
- Make it EASY to BEHAVE in the desired way by starting out so small that there's no reason to not do it, such as just sitting in the meditation area for ten seconds.
- Make the REWARD SATISFACTORY by compiling a list of the benefits you'll get from regular meditation and displaying it somewhere you'll see it regularly.

When you're in the process of changing habits, it's best to focus on one at a time. Give yourself permission to start out small and, as we discussed in the S.T.E.P.S Formula, there is NO start that is too small. In fact, you want to make the start SO small that you can't possibly say no to it. Once you're successfully doing that super small thing consistently, then you can layer on the habit over time.

Another way to make it easier is to attach it to something that you already do, which then becomes the CUE or TRIGGER. Create a statement around it, such as:

"When I _____, I will _____."

Let's apply this to the example of creating a meditation habit, which is actually a real example from my own life. I wanted to meditate on a daily basis, but it just wasn't happening. I was very inconsistent. So, I started by creating a meditation corner in a part of my house that I had to walk past every single morning, making it VISIBLE. I put a comfy chair and little table in there. I put a colourful mat on the floor and a lovely tablecloth on the table. I added my Oracle cards, crystals, candles, and a lamp that I loved, making it so ATTRACTIVE that I wanted to spend time there. My normal daily routine was that I would get up, get dressed, and then go downstairs to go about my day, and I had to walk past my meditation corner to go downstairs, so I decided to attach my meditation habit to getting dressed in the morning. My CUE or TRIGGER was getting dressed in the morning and then I would start with sitting in my meditation chair for just ten seconds.

The statement I created was:

"When I get dressed in the morning, I will sit in my meditation chair for ten seconds."

That's it. No expectation to do ANY meditation. Just sit in my meditation chair for ten seconds. Why? Because who can say no to ten seconds?

It didn't matter if I got up late, if I had a lot to do, or whatever else was going on, I could always find ten seconds. By creating the meditation corner in a place where I had to walk past it and making the first step so small that I couldn't say no, I was making it EASY to behave in the way that I wanted, and I had done research on the benefits of meditation, so the REWARD was SATISFACTORY to me.

For the next week, after I got dressed in the morning, I would happily go and sit in my meditation chair for ten seconds. The habit was so small that there was absolutely no way that I could say no to doing it and this is a critical success key to creating a new habit. The even more awesome thing that happened was once I sat in my meditation chair, I would always do a small meditation, even if it was only for a minute. I was already in the chair, so why not? There was no expectation, but I did it, which was a win, and also another helpful strategy that we will go into later.

The next week I started to layer on my new habit. My new statement was:

"When I get dressed in the morning, I will sit in my meditation chair and meditate for at least one minute."

I would keep track of my success and if I managed to perform the habit at least five out of seven days, then I would layer again. The next week, I increased the meditation to two minutes, then the next week three minutes, and so on until I got to six minutes.

The habit was now created and at least five days out of seven, after I got dressed in the morning, I would sit in my meditation chair and meditate for however much time I had on that day. There is not one day that I sat in that chair that I couldn't do at least one minute of meditation and that made me feel really good because even one minute of meditation five days a week is better than none.

Meditation habit successfully created!

What If Your Habit Isn't Forming?

So, what happens if the habit you're trying to create isn't happening? That's when you need to start examining each of the four elements:

- The CUE or TRIGGER
- The DESIRE
- The BEHAVIOUR
- The REWARD

Is the CUE or TRIGGER the right one? If you aren't a morning person, it's not the best idea to create a morning exercise habit. Instead, try attaching it to something later in the day.

If changing the CUE or TRIGGER doesn't work, then assess if the DESIRE is ATTRACTIVE enough. Do you WANT to do it? This comes back to PLEASURABLE from the S.T.E.P.S Formula.

You could then look at whether the issue is the BEHAVIOUR that you're trying to create. Are you trying to take too big a step to soon? If you're a busy mum trying to create a yoga habit in the morning, whilst five minutes may not seem like a long time, it could be too long in the initiation phase.

If you're not successfully initiating the habit, and the CUE or TRIGGER seems ok, then try decreasing the size of the habit from five minutes of yoga to just doing a single yoga pose. Once you're doing that consistently, then layer on it to two yoga poses and so on until you get to the yoga session duration you're aiming for.

Finally, if the CUE or TRIGGER and the BEHAVIOUR seem ok, then analyse the REWARD element. Is the REWARD big enough for you to go out of your way to achieve it? If not, then you won't be able to create a long-term habit.

A final strategy to help wire in a habit quicker is to perform the habit five times over seven days, creating a chain. Each time you perform the habit, congratulate yourself and celebrate. When your brain associates performing the habit with positive emotions, it wires it in.

Your Organic Story

What's the story you're telling yourself when it comes to switching to organic? Are you telling yourself that it's too hard? That you can't afford it? Instead, tell yourself that you're resourceful and can find a way to do it within your budget. Remind yourself that you're CHOOSING to make the switch because you want better health and longevity. Change the story to "I'm worth the investment."

Finding Support

The biggest gift you can give yourself on this journey is the gift of support. This could be support from family and friends, apps or other resources, like-minded communities, coaching or education, or a myriad of different things. Give yourself the gift of lots of support and ask for help when you need it.

If you haven't already joined our Facebook Group (shariware.com/BME), jump in and introduce yourself and say Hi!

Your Organic Blueprint Action Step

Before you start, watch this short video
(shariware.com/YOBASChapter2) to get some tips on how to
get the most out of this action step.

- On **Page 5** of your downloadable workbook, do the
  "Finding Your WHY" exercise for your switch to
  organic.

- Once you've found your WHY POWER! jump into our
  Facebook Group (shariware.com/BME) and share
  whatever you feel comfortable sharing.

"

"If your WHY doesn't make you CRY, it's not strong enough!"

-shari ware

Chapter 3
Goals For Your Organic Lifestyle

Now we get to have some fun! This is where you get to be creative and design what you want Your Organic Blueprint to look like. Are you excited? Let's do it!

When it comes to achieving goals in your life, it's essential to identify two important points:

1. The end goal or destination
2. Where you currently are or where you're starting from.

In this chapter, you're going to focus on the destination and ask yourself the following questions (there will be an action step at the end of the chapter to delve into these further):

- Where is the destination you want to get to?
- What does your destination look like?
- What does it feel like at your destination?
- How will you know you have arrived at your destination?
- Is anyone coming on the journey with you?
- Think about how you feel after arriving at your destination. On a scale of 1-10 (where 1 is not good and 10 is amazing), how would you rate it?
- Write down three words to describe how you'll feel once you have arrived at your destination.

This isn't about the steps you need to take to get there or any of the nitty gritty stuff. This is a "perfect world" scenario. The sky is the limit and it's about allowing your mind to go to wherever it wants to go.

Your Organic Blueprint Action Step

Before you start, watch this short video (shariware.com/YOBASChapter3) to get some tips on how to get the most out of this action step.

Focus on the destination and ask yourself the following questions on **Page 7** of your downloadable workbook:

- Where is the destination you want to get to?
- What does your destination look like?
- What does it feel like at your destination?
- How will you know you have arrived at your destination?
- Is anyone coming on the journey with you?
- Thinking about how you feel after arriving at your destination. On a scale of 1-10 (where 1 is not good and 10 is amazing), how would you rate it?
- Write down three words to describe how you'll feel once you have arrived at your destination.

66

"Aim for the stars. Even if you don't make it all the way, you're still up!"

—shari ware

Chapter 4
Assessing Your Current Lifestyle

> Now that you know where you're going, you need to know where you are. This chapter is all about assessing where you are now so you can plan your journey to get to your end destination.

Imagine that you're driving somewhere you haven't been before. These days, you plug the address into a GPS, and it guides you to your destination. For that to happen, though, the GPS also must have the starting location.

This situation is no different. Whenever you set yourself a goal in life, not only do you need to know your destination, but you also need to know where you are.

So where are you? In this chapter, you're going to focus on your starting point and ask yourself the following questions (just consider these for now and, as in the previous chapter, there will be an action step at the end to delve into them further):

- Where are you now?
- What does it look like where you are?
- What does it feel like where you are?
- Thinking about how you feel now. On a scale of 1-10 (where 1 is not good and 10 is amazing), how would you rate it?
- Write down three words to describe how you feel now.

Again, this is not about the steps you need to take to get there or any of the nitty gritty stuff. We'll get to that in the next chapter. Before we get to that though, you have some action steps to take!

Your Organic Blueprint Action Step

Before you start, watch this short video (shariware.com/YOBASChapter4) to get some tips on how to get the most out of this action step.

Focus on your starting point and ask yourself the following questions on **Page 9** of your downloadable workbook:

- Where are you now?
- What does it look like where you are?
- What does it feel like where you are?
- Thinking about how you feel now. On a scale of 1-10 (where 1 is not good and 10 is amazing), how would you rate it?
- Write down three words to describe how you feel now.

66

"Where you are now is just a point on your journey that will show you which way you need to go."

-shari ware

Chapter 5

Navigating the Maze: Practical & Budget-Friendly Tips

> Now it's time for the nitty gritty stuff. I know that you were probably wondering if we were ever going to get here, and we have finally arrived!

Now that you're clear on your destination and where you're starting from, it's time to plan your journey. Having a look at the GPS, you can see there are a few different routes to your destination. One way may be a bit shorter in time, one might be a more direct route, one will take you over a toll road, and one might be the scenic drive.

This chapter is about deciding which way you're going to go to reach your destination and will help you begin creating Your Organic Blueprint. Ask yourself the following questions (just consider these for now and, as in the previous chapters, there will be an action step at the end to delve into them further):

- How are you going to get to your destination?
- What do you want to change?
- Are you on a budget?
- Are you bringing anyone else along for the ride?
- Can you foresee any obstacles or challenges?

Now we'll discuss some practical tools, tips, and strategies that will help you to navigate the journey through the maze painlessly and effortlessly. Are we there yet? (Pun intended!) As in, do you believe that the transition can be painless and effortless? Maybe you're not quite all the way to believing me yet, but you will be after this chapter, so strap on your seatbelt and let's go!

When it comes to actually making the transition to organic, it can seem overwhelming and difficult to decide where to start. You may want to go through your entire house and throw out anything that you feel is not the healthiest and replace it all in one hit, or you might want to do it more slowly, especially if budget is an issue or if doing it in one hit feels overwhelming, which is where I was at.

So, let's set some ground rules for the physical transition. Firstly, there is no right or wrong way to do anything. This is YOUR journey, and you do whatever is "EASYest" (remember S.T.E.P.S!) for YOU.

Secondly, apply the S.T.E.P.S Formula to EVERYTHING. Focus on one SMALL change at a time and give yourself a quick win by choosing the "EASYest" change to make first. This is a marathon, not a sprint (an oldie but a goodie!) and Rome wasn't built in a day (corny but relevant!).

Hands up the perfectionists in the room! If this is you, then please check your perfectionist hat at the door. This advice comes from a recovering perfectionist – me, myself and I. It's not about being perfect, it's about being a little bit better every day.

B ME – Better Me Every Day!

In keeping with this premise, it doesn't have to be "organic" right away, just "better". Any better choice is progress in the direction of a healthier you.

And last but definitely not least, remember at the beginning of the book I said that there was one belief that I was right about? Well, it's coming right up and it's something that you just have to make peace with to be able to make this transition painless and effortless.

You'll Never Be Done!
Mic drop!

Just let that sink in for a moment. You might have already figured it out and that's awesome. I know it's something that I struggled with in the beginning though, and so it's best to just rip that band-aid off and get it out in the open if you're not on the same page.

There's no way it CAN ever be done, and you just have to be ok with that and "let it go" (can you hear Elsa singing? Sorry, not sorry!).

There are so many things that you have no control over, and you'll literally drive yourself batty trying to look at every little thing that you could ever change. Life wouldn't be much fun and what would be the point of it all?

If you're embarking on this journey, then you probably want a healthier you and you won't achieve that by stressing yourself out over the multitude of things that you haven't changed. Focus on being a little bit better every day and know that ANY better choice is better than zero better choices.

Now that we've got the ground rules set, let's talk about some of the options for sourcing organic products, including some that are more budget friendly.

Organic Labels
Just because something is labelled "Organic" or "Certified Organic" doesn't mean that it's better. The term "Organic" can sometimes just mean that it contains organic material, not that

said organic material is free from chemicals and pesticides, either in whole or part.

When it comes to "Certified Organic", some companies closely imitate wording or logos to make something appear as if it is certified organic when it isn't. For example, a product might say "organically certified" but not actually have the organic certification. Before you get started on your journey, ensure that you know the legitimate wording and logos for certified organic products in your country.

Also, the process to become certified organic involves a lot of money and red tape and some businesses just don't have the resources to be able to get the formal certification, but they are actually organic, so be on the lookout for them and ask if you're not sure.

Fresh Produce

When you're looking for fresh produce, you'll generally find the best quality and the most budget-friendly options at the local farmers market, local farms, or natural co-ops. Some will be Certified Organic, but some may not be. Also be on the lookout for "Spray Free" – these are generally farmers that don't use chemicals but haven't gone down the path of getting certified organic accreditation.

If you don't know where your local markets are, you can look them up online. They're usually on the weekends and it makes a nice outing each week to pop down and get your local produce. You also get the bonus of human connection, vitamin D from getting out in the sun, and a great feeling knowing that you're supporting local farmers and small businesses, so it's a win, win, win, win!

36

If you're on a budget and want to keep costs down, some fresh produce items aren't so bad if you can't get organic, including anything with a thick skin that you're not going to eat, such as watermelon or avocados. Produce that is "in season" will also be cheaper.

The Dirty Dozen

The following list is called "The Dirty Dozen" and includes the produce with the highest contamination from pesticides, according to the Environmental Working Group (EWG). You definitely want to buy organic for any of the following:

- Strawberries
- Spinach
- Kale, Collard, and Mustard Greens
- Peaches
- Pears
- Nectarines
- Apples
- Grapes
- Bell & Hot Peppers
- Cherries
- Blueberries
- Green Beans

Below is a list of items called "The Clean Fifteen", which are the produce with the least contamination from pesticides according to the EWG. If you need to bring your budget into balance, these are the ones that you might choose to skimp on. If you do and you're not peeling and throwing the skin away, then give them a wash in filtered water and baking soda to remove any chemical residue:

- Avocados

- Sweet Corn
- Pineapple
- Onions
- Papaya
- Sweet Peas (Frozen)
- Asparagus
- Honeydew Melon
- Kiwi Fruit
- Cabbage
- Mushrooms
- Mangoes
- Sweet Potatoes
- Watermelon
- Carrots

Some other things you can do to keep the cost down are:

- Grow your own fresh produce.
- Buy in-season produce and freeze it, dehydrate it, or preserve it.

Meat

Look around for local, organic, grass-fed farmers to buy your meat from. It will be cheaper because they don't have to pay for refrigerated transport. Ask your farmers if their animals are 100% grass fed and whether they use antibiotics. Even if the farmer doesn't have organic certification, if they only feed their animals grass and they don't use antibiotics, then they are a great source for you to buy your meat. You'll generally have to purchase either a whole, half or quarter of a beast, which means you'll need a lot of freezer room, or you can split it with friends. You'll pay a whole lot less this way though.

Next, find an organic butcher. They are few and far between, but if you live in a populated area, there will be one somewhere, even if you have to go a little out of your way, it's worth it. Their prices will generally range from mid to high and some price points may be out of your budget, so keep the cost down by buying the cheaper cuts.

I currently buy the cheaper cuts from an organic butcher. They are a 30-minute drive from where I live, so we do a weekly shop scheduled for when we're already going to be in the area. We also get our fresh produce from the same area, so before we come home, we get our fruit and veg from our organic fresh produce supplier.

If you're shopping in the grocery store, look for organic, grass-fed, or free-range meat or poultry and wild caught seafood.

Another way to keep the cost down is to spread the meat out and bulk meals up with more vegetables. Our daily protein requirements are only 150g – 210g per day, so sticking to that will help. Make stews, casseroles, and curries with lots of veggies and keep any bones to make bone broth. You can even incorporate one or two "meat free" days per week if you really want to cut down on your budget.

Other Grocery Items

Eggs are a big one to watch out for. Organic and free range are what you're looking for here. They are a great source of protein so if you're cutting your meat portions, you can add some eggs into the mix. The best place to get them at a decent price is generally your local farmers market, co-op, or straight from the farm.

If you're in the grocery store and looking at the price range on eggs, organic free range will be at the top of the range, and most

39

probably $5-$6 more than the cheapest ones. When you're first starting to transition, I know that can be a BIG step and it's something that I personally struggled with.

I reminded myself that firstly, the chickens laying the eggs were much happier because they weren't crammed into a cage with other chickens and lived a much happier life, which means the eggs produced are higher quality and much more nourishing for my body than eggs produced from chickens that live in high-stress and inhumane conditions.

Secondly and equally, I told myself that I was worth the investment in my health. I had to do that a LOT in the beginning, but now it has become a habit that I don't question and I always get the best quality eggs that I can regardless of the price. I still shop around to see where I can get the same quality cheaper, though!

Organic on a Budget
If you have a Costco near you, you can find a good range of organic products at cheaper prices than you would find in a normal grocery store.

When it comes to shopping on a budget, one of the best things you can do is to meal plan beforehand. Do your weekly, fortnightly, or monthly meal plan, depending on how often you shop and then create your shopping list. This will help you utilize what you already have in the pantry and ensure that you're only buying what you need for the period you're shopping for, which will help you stay within your budget. It also helps with making sure you're using up what you have in your pantry, so it gets rotated and doesn't go to waste. Win-win!

If you're shopping in a standard grocery store, you'll find a lot of organic or better choices. It's all about reading labels, which we

40

will talk about more in depth in the next chapter. I will also tell you about some apps that can show which products are ok and which ones to avoid. Before we get to that though, it's time to take another action step!

Your Organic Blueprint Action Step

Before you start, watch this short video (shariware.com/YOBASChapter5) to get some tips on how to get the most out of this action step.

This action step is about deciding which way you're going to go to reach your destination and the beginning of creating **Your Organic Blueprint**. Answer the following questions on **Page 11** of your downloadable workbook:

- How are you going to get to your destination?
- What do you want to change?
- Are you on a budget?
- Are you bringing anyone else along for the ride?
- Can you foresee any obstacles or challenges?

Once you've done the exercise, jump into the Facebook Group (shariware.com/BME) and share whatever you feel comfortable sharing, specifically any challenges that you've identified so that we can help you with solutions!

"Many small changes add up to a massive transformation in the end."

-shari ware

Chapter 6
In Plain Sight: Reading Ingredient Labels

This is one of the most important chapters in the book and by the end of it, you'll know how to better identify which products are good for you and which are best to avoid. It's amazing what can be hidden in plain sight on a product label!

The first thing you need to know about labels is that the best foods don't have them. The second thing to know about labels is that it's important to study them when they're there.

The smaller the ingredient list, the better – one or two organic ingredients on the list is wonderful and means you're less likely to find nasties hiding somewhere. The longer the list, the more likely it is there will be something in there that isn't great.

The order is also important. The ingredients are listed in the percentage order, with the highest first. So, if you have a product where sugar (or a form of sugar) is the first or second ingredient on the list, then that product is made up of a whole lot of sugar. Whilst organic sugar may be better than non-organic, sugar is sugar and best eaten in small quantities.

Sugar
There are over 70 different names for sugar that can be found on ingredient lists and it can be hidden in products that you wouldn't even think would have sugar in it, such as salad dressing. On a food label, sugar could be listed as:

- Sugar, brown sugar, palm sugar, etc.
- Anything ending in "ose".

- Maple syrup, brown rice syrup, malt syrup, etc.
- Honey, agave, molasses, etc.

Artificial sweeteners and sugar substitutes aren't necessarily better and can often be worse, especially when they aren't natural. Be on the lookout for artificial sweeteners like sucralose, aspartame, acesulfame potassium, or saccharin.

It's also important to be aware of sugar alcohols which end in "-ol" such as xylitol, erythritol, mannitol, lactitol, sorbitol or malititol, as well as synthethic sweeteners produced from natural ingredients like stevia and monk fruit extract.

Fats & Oils
Unhealthy fats and oils are another thing to look out for. A product high in trans fats is best left on the shelf. "Oils 'aint oils" and all that jazz, so steering clear of products that contain seed oils such as canola oil, grapeseed oil, and sunflower oil is preferable.

Olive oil is one of the best choices in my opinion, and something that I personally use a lot of.

Additives, Preservatives & Artificial Colours
Some product labels are made up of a whole lot of numbers. These are the additives, preservatives, and artificial colours and flavourings. As with anything, some are worse than others, but it's best to reduce consumption of anything that has a number or list of numbers in the ingredient list.

Wood Pulp & Petroleum
Why are we talking about these? Because you can find them in processed foods. Petrol in food? Yup. How can it be ok to put petrol in food you ask? I don't have an answer for you. I was gob-smacked and horrified when I found out. But somehow, it's

ok and so you have to do your due diligence and find it yourself, so you don't unwittingly consume it in some way.

Let's start with wood pulp. This has a few different names on an ingredient list, including:

- Cellulose
- Cellulose gum
- Cellulose gel
- Microcrystalline cellulose (MCC)
- Or the more technical term, carboxymethyl cellulose

It's used as an anti-caking agent and its commonly added to grated cheese to stop it sticking together. According to some sources, it's not harmful, but it's up to you to make the decision on that and now that you're aware of it, you can.

Now let's talk about petroleum. You would be surprised at what foods it's found in. It's quite often labelled as "mineral oil" and can be found in packaged baked products to stop them from spoiling and canned goods to extend shelf life. You'll also find it in chicken nuggets, rice crackers, frozen pizzas, and cookies.

A lot of food colourings and food additives contain petroleum derivatives and they are added to a myriad of products from fruit snacks to drinks to corn chips. Some chocolates are even made with food-grade parrafin wax. Petrochemicals can also quite often be found in vitamins and pain killers such as aspirin.

The following is a list of names for petroleum that you might find on a food label:

- Butylated hydroxyanisole (BHA)
- Ethyl methylphenidate
- Methyl benzoate

- Mineral oil
- Parrafin Wax
- Tertiary butylhydroquinone (TBHQ)
- Tert-butylhydroquinone (TBHQ)
- Blue 1
- Blue 2
- Red 40
- Yellow 5
- Yellow 6

As you can see, there is so much that can be hiding in plain sight on a food label and now you're much better equipped to be able to pick the good from the bad.

Food Label Apps

There are some great apps that you can download to your phone which allow you to scan products to find out if they're a good choice or something that would be best left on the shelf.

My personal favourites are "Think Dirty" and "Yuka – Food and Cosmetic Scanner". Now it's time to check out some labels!

Your Organic Blueprint Action Step

Download **Think Dirty** or **Yuka** (or both) and go to your kitchen to have a look at the labels of at least five products that you use regularly. If there are any that have ingredients that you don't recognize, scan them to see if they're good or not so good choices.

- On **Page 13** of your downloadable workbook, write down any products that aren't good and that you want to find a healthier swap for.

Next time you go shopping, look for a better option for those particular products.

> "The most important thing to remember about food labels is that the best foods have none."

— shari ware

Chapter 7
Celebrating Your Organic Journey

Congratulations are in order! It's time to celebrate you and how far you've come. Even just by reading this book and doing the action steps, you have made progress towards your destination.

Yes, you're at the beginning of your journey and the destination may seem a long way away, but I promise that if you continue taking one Small, Timely, Easy, Pleasurable, Sustainable step at a time, you'll get there.

Remember the car analogy? This is what I remind my clients of constantly and I want to remind you of it now. You're in your car, you're strapped in and good to go. You put the GPS on, the voice tells you where to go and you're off! Along the way, you need a toilet break, and you have to make a stop. When you're back on the road, you come across some roadworks and have to slow down and then you have to take a detour. Further down the road, you miss a turn and have to turn around and go back. You hit some speed bumps and potholes on the way, and you have to make another stop to get petrol because your fuel light comes on.

Eventually though, you finally arrive at your destination. You may not have gotten there the way you thought you would or as fast as you might have liked, but you did get there in the end. You always do. The only time you don't is when you decide it's all too hard and turn around and go home.

Remember that this journey is just like getting in a car and driving to a new destination. You'll get there, as long as you keep going. It doesn't matter if there are some detours, wrong turns, or speed bumps along the way. What matters is that you get there.

So, give yourself a high five, a pat on the back, a massive hug, and tell yourself how amazing you are, because you are!

In Chapter 8, I'm going to share with you some of the things that I have changed or implemented in my life that could help you, but before we move on to that, it's time for you to reflect on wins that you have made thus far. Just consider the following and at the end of the chapter, there will be an action step for you to do (of course!):

- What are the three biggest WINS you've gained from reading this book that will help you on your journey moving forward?
- Thinking about how you feel NOW about the difficulty of transitioning to organic AFTER reading this book. On a scale of 1-10 (where 1 is difficult and 10 is easy), how would you rate it?
- Write down three words to describe how you NOW feel about the difficulty of transitioning to organic.

Your Organic Blueprint Action Step

Before you start, watch this short video (shariware.com/YOBASChapter7) to get some tips on how to get the most out of this action step.

On **Page 14** of your downloadable workbook, answer the following questions:

- What are the three biggest WINS you've gained from reading this book that will help you in your journey moving forward?
- Thinking about how you feel NOW about the difficulty of transitioning to organic AFTER reading this book. On a scale of 1-10 (where 1 is difficult and 10 is easy), how would you rate it?
- Write down three words to describe how you NOW feel about the difficulty of transitioning to organic.

Once you've completed the action step, share your three biggest WINS in the Facebook Group (shariware.com/BME) so that we can all celebrate you!

"Remember to celebrate the distance you have already traveled."

-shari ware

Chapter 8
Shari's Suggestions

In this chapter, I'll share with you some of the things I've switched in my own home and resources I use that I have found helpful. There are lots of options out there and it can be helpful to have some strategies that you know someone else has tried and tested.

Below is a list of resources that I have found helpful, along with important items that I have switched in my own home and budget-friendly alternatives. You'll find a list of the relevant links to check them all out on **Page 16** of your downloadable workbook.

Apps
- Think Dirty
- Yuka – Food and Cosmetic Scanner

Groceries
You can find a variety of organic items at **Costco** that are budget friendly. Buy in bulk and save some dollars!

Water, Water, Water!
If you're drinking tap water, then you definitely want to prioritise switching your water source. There are lots of great options out there, but I chose the **Alps Water Filter**, which I consider to be one of the greatest investments I have ever made. I love my Alps Water Filter because not only does it take the nasties out of my water, but it adds back in good stuff as it goes through the filtration system.

Essential Oils

I make a lot of my own cleaning products with vinegar and essential oils. I also use essential oils as perfume and my daughter makes her furbaby's shampoo and adds essential oils to it as well. Not all essential oils are pet-friendly though, so it's important to check before you use an essential oil for your pet or for floors, surfaces, etc.

Not all essential oils are of the same quality and the brand I love the most are **Doterra Oils**.

Heavy Metal Detox

As well as switching to chemical free, I highly recommend doing a heavy metal detox. Your body will love you for it!

Heavy metal toxicity can cause chronic mental health issues, fatigue, nausea, brain fog, migraines or headaches, digestive problems, and the list goes on. Heavy metals can be found in our water, household products, farmed fish and dental fillings. They penetrate various organ and tissue cells in our body and can be stored there for years.

By switching to organic and reducing processed foods as much as possible you're already helping your body to detox heavy metals. Changing your water as previously discussed will also help greatly and the Alps Water Filter that I suggested has the added benefit of **Zeolite**, which is great for detoxing heavy metals. There are also Zeolite supplements that you can take that give your body that extra helping hand that it needs.

The Environmental Working Group (EWG)

The Environmental Working Group is the organization that publishes The Dirty Dozen and The Clean Fifteen and updates them annually. You'll find links to them on **Page 17** of your downloadable workbook.

Fresh Produce

If you want to start growing your own nutrient-dense, organic produce and you have no idea where to start, then I highly recommend **The Healthy Patch**. Their program shows you how to build your own chemical-free, raised garden beds to grow organic, nutrient-dense food all year round. No matter what climate you live in, you'll get step-by-step advice, and no previous gardening experience is necessary.

Food for Your Pets

Just like you're looking for better options for yourself, remember to look for better options for your furbaby. My daughter and I realized that our furbaby Lulu wasn't getting all the nutrients that she needed from the raw mince that she was being fed. After doing some research, we decided to give **Frontier Pets** a try. Lulu loves it and we know that she is getting everything she needs, so win-win!

Blue Light

Blue light at night impacts your Circadian rhythm in a big way and reducing it as much as possible will benefit you greatly. If you're looking at screens at night, I highly recommend **Blue Light Blocking Glasses** and downloading a free software called **f.lux** to your computer to reduce the blue light.

You can also put your phone or tablet on "Night Shift", and it will automatically reduce the blue light emitted from your phone between the hours that you set. Another thing you can do is have **salt lamps** around your home and turn them on at night instead of white lights.

Wi-Fi/EMF/Radiation

High levels of EMF exposure can be harmful to your health. Turning your Wi-Fi off at night is a great way to reduce levels. There are also lots of EMF Reducing Products on the market and I am slowly implementing them in my home, starting with putting **EMF neutralizer stickers** on my devices.

Filtrating Plants

One of the easiest, most inexpensive ways to improve the air quality in your home is by adding plants wherever you can. I have **potted plants** in the main living areas of my home and in the bedrooms. One of the best plants you can have in the bedroom is Snake Plant (AKA Mother in Law's Tongue) because it filters toxins from the air.

My Effortlessly Organic Program

There are many facets to switching to a non-toxic lifestyle and way too many to put in this book. That would be another way to send you into overwhelm. This book is a bite-size chunk designed to give you really strong foundations on which to build Your Organic Blueprint. This is the first step on your journey to a more natural lifestyle and once you've finished it, it's time for step two.

My **Effortlessly Organic Program** will help you cement in a lot of the tools and strategies outlined in this book. It will also help you to refine Your Organic Blueprint further and you'll delve deeper into areas that we haven't explored fully in this book.

If you're keen to find out more, you'll find details on **Page 19** of your downloadable workbook.

I really hope that you have received value from this book and that it will be a great resource for you moving forward. One of the extra awesome things is that almost everything in this book can be applied across every aspect of your life for anything that you want to change. It doesn't matter what change you want to make, if you apply these same principles, it will be a whole lot easier!

About The Author

Shari Ware is a beacon for those seeking to navigate the path towards a healthier, more organic way of living. With a personal story that resonates with transformation and perseverance, Shari embodies the journey from a challenging weight loss endeavour in 2010 to an inspiring realisation in 2016 that true health encompasses making organic and mindful lifestyle choices.

Facing the same doubts and hurdles that many encounter—the costs, the time, the overwhelming nature of big lifestyle changes—Shari overcame these and evolved, not just in her personal health but in her mission to guide others. She has proven that it's not only possible to enhance one's health and that of your family while adhering to one's core principles, but that it's also achievable on a budget and within a busy schedule.

The cornerstone of Shari's philosophy is the S.T.E.P.S Formula, an approach grounded in the practical application of neuroscience designed to be economically feasible. She stands as an unwavering pillar of support for those she guides, valuing honesty above all in her efforts to keep it authentic and real.

Shari's message is one of relentless positivity and realistic expectations: perfection is not the goal on this journey, but rather, the continuous striving for personal improvement. She encourages embracing the twists and turns of one's unique path with no judgment on the pace or direction of progress.

As the driving force behind the B ME Movement, Shari Ware invites everyone to join in the collective goal of becoming a Better Me Every Day while still Being Me!, fostering a community dedicated to the pursuit of a more wholesome, organic lifestyle.

If you would like to connect, please reach out to me on Facebook (https://shariware.com/BME)

I hope you enjoyed this book. Please feel free to share it with friends and post a review so I can help more people to be a little better every day!

Shari Ware

xoxo

www.ingramcontent.com/pod-product-compliance
Lightning Source LLC
Chambersburg PA
CBHW041301040426
42334CB00028BA/3120